I0085989

THE TALES OF MY WEED

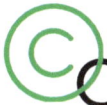

© Charles R Haffner and RJ Tungsten 2024

ISBN: 978-0-7961-8496-2

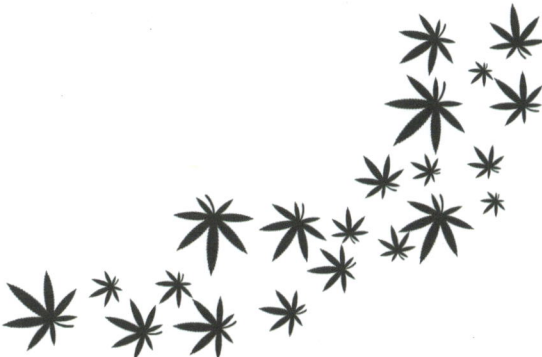

ABOUT THIS BOOK

The Tales of My Weed is a poetic collection that ranges from Haiku to Cinquain. These wonderful stories highlight and celebrate the 420 smoking life.

A unique perspective from the minds of Charles Haffner and RJ Tungsten paying homage to the plant they enjoy and respect so much.

The works inside are from the past, present, and soon-to-be future. So get comfortable and enjoy your favorite munchies as you journey through some high tales.

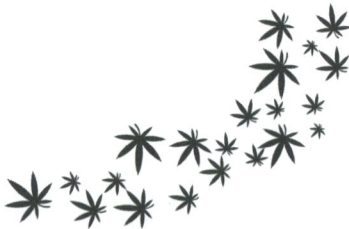

ABOUT THE AUTHORS

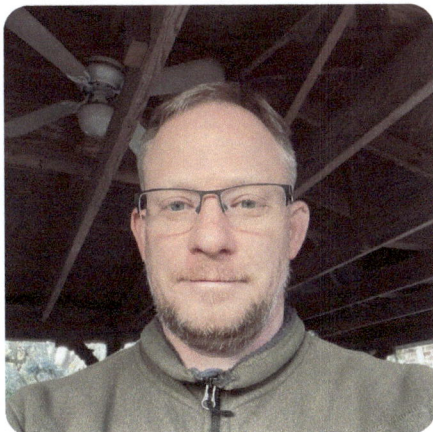

ABOUT 5 YEARS AGO RJ TUNGSTEN NOTICED HE HAD A CREATIVE SIDE. IT CAME IN THE FORM OF HAIKU POETRY. HE ENJOYS THE CHALLENGE OF THE WORD PUZZLE AND CAPTURING A MOMENT IN TIME. HIS WORKS HAVE BEEN PUBLISHED ALL OVER THE WORLD. RJ LIVES IN CHARLESTON SOUTH CAROLINA

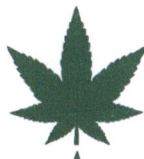

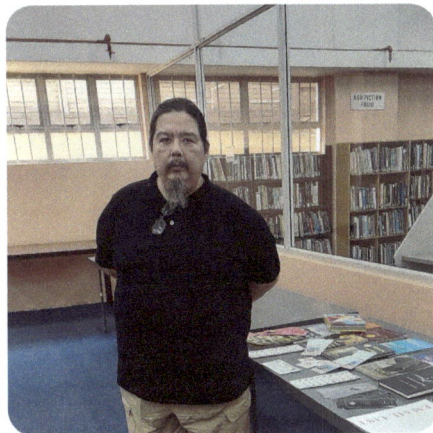

CHARLES R HAFFNER WAS BORN IN BALTIMORE MARYLAND AND LIVED IN CENTRAL FLORIDA FOR 15 YEARS. FOR THE PAST TWO YEARS, HE HAS WRITTEN 9 BOOKS CONSISTING OF VARIOUS FORMS OF MICRO POETRY. HIS BOOKS CAN BE FOUND ON AMAZON.COM AND HE IS THE CO-OWNER OF SAKURA BOOK PUBLISHING. HE RESIDES IN SOUTH AFRICA.

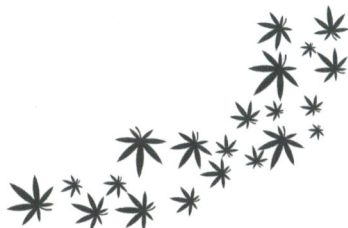

GRINDED OR SPLIT UP
MATERIAL LOOKS MATTER
ALSO FOR FUNCTION.

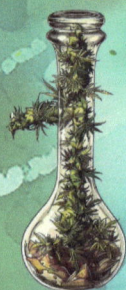

SITTING ROUND' FIRE
BOWL SPARKED AND PASSED TO THE LEFT
STORIES FILL THE AIR.

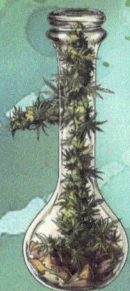

SOME WHAT SPACED YET COMPLETELY GROUNDED STATE OF BEING IN MY FOG.

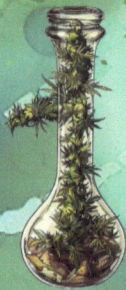

MUSIC HITS HARDER
DEVILS LETTUCE ENHANCEMENT
COMPLETELY ZONED IN.

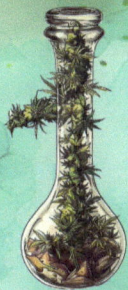

NIGHTLY RITUAL
ENJOY THE SETUP CLEAN UP
AND THE IN BETWEEN.

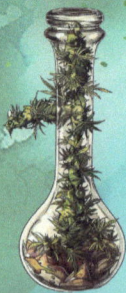

GRIND THE DENSITY
MOST IMPRESSIVE YIELD OF SHAKE
COMBUSTION GOODNESS

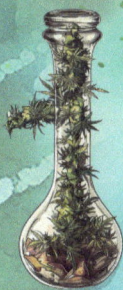

THE PINCH FROM NATURE
EARTH'S BOUNTY SHARED WITH MANKIND
A SELFLESS GIFTING.

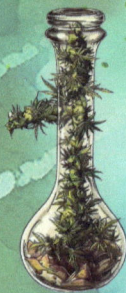

FIRE SPARKED GOODNESS
TAKE ME ON AN ADVENTURE
OPENS MY THIRD EYE.

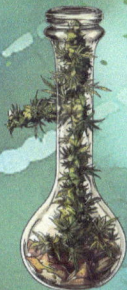

TAKE A HIT AND PASS
ABSORB ALL THE MEDICINE
REAP THE BENEFITS.

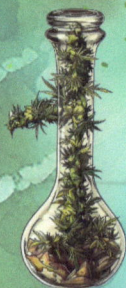

SKILLFUL BOTANY
PRECISION ENGINEERING
DEGREES MADE FROM WEED.

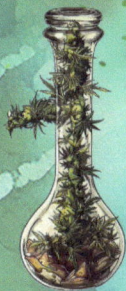

ALUMINUM CAN
MAYBE A GREEN APPLE CORE
ROOKIE DEVICES.

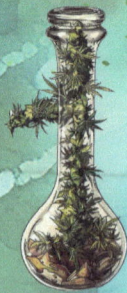

NICKEL BAG OR DIME
HOW ABOUT WE GET SOME WEIGHT
MAKE IT LAST THIS TIME.

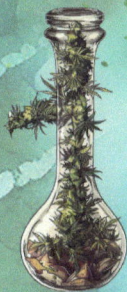

HOTBOXING WITH FRIENDS
PARK THE CAR IN A SAFE PLACE
WHO BLOCKED THE DRIVEWAY?

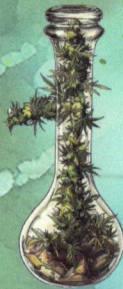

ATTEMPT A NEW WAY
CUT THE TOP OFF A BOTTLE
BONG OF GRAVITY.

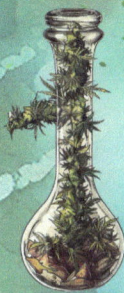

ALL THE STASH IS GONE
NECESSARY ADVENTURE
WATCH OUT FOR THE COPS.

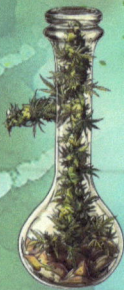

ROLL IT
LOVE THE PROCESS
INHALING THE GOODNESS
INDICA OR SATISFACTION
WE'RE HIGH.

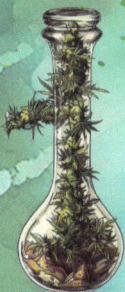

PRE ROLL FIRED UP
ADDED A VAPE IN THE MIX
DEEP CONVERSATION.

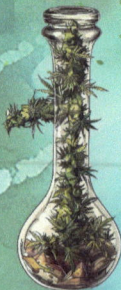

NEW TECHNOLOGY
HOW DO WE TURN THIS THING ON?
BUTTON CLICKED FIVE TIMES
APPARENTLY NEEDED COLLEGE
DEGREE TO GET HIGH TODAY.

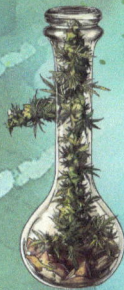

THANKS FOR THE GREAT NIGHT
IT'S LATE, GONNA HEAD HOME NOW
LOOKS LIKE A MISSED TURN
JUST HAD TO TAKE THAT LAST HIT
NAVIGATION HELP NEEDED

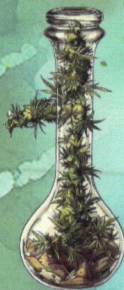

PASSION

GREEN ENHANCEMENT

COMING TOGETHER NOW

SHARING THE CUSTOMARY SPLIFF

ONENESS.

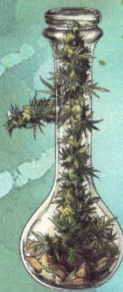

SMOKE INDUCED COUCH LOCK
HOW DID I GET HERE? CAN'T LEAVE!
PERMA GRIN PASTED

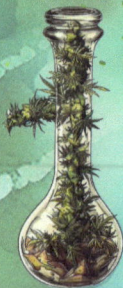

COLLEGE HOUSE HANG OUT
SOMEONE BROKE OUT THE MUSHROOMS
MAIL JUST THEN ARRIVED
A CARE PACKAGE FROM CALI
CONCOCTION OF GOODNESS SMOKED.

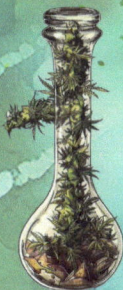

SEA BREEZE HITS MY FACE
CANNABIS SWIRLS IN MY LUNGS
MATCH MADE IN HEAVEN

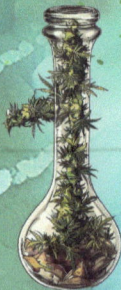

BLUNTED TEENAGER
EMBARKING ON FAST FOOD
ADVENTURE WITH MY FRIENDS
MEMORY FRIED FOR SHORT TERM
LET'S PAY AND FORGET THE FOOD.

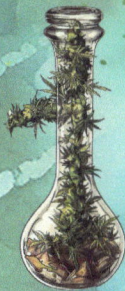

LET'S SHOTGUN A HIT
A HOPEFUL REQUEST TO THE
PRETTY GIRL PRESENT.

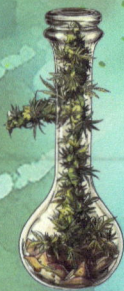

**INTERNATIONAL
TIME TO GET HIGH HAS APPROACHED
IT'S 4:20 NOW.**

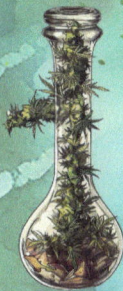

WAKE AND BAKE ACTION
GETTING THE DAY STARTED RIGHT
BIG YAWN, IT'S NAP TIME.

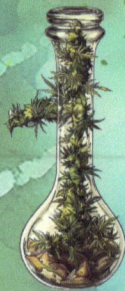

A WONDERFUL FLOWER I CAN SMOKE.
GRIND IT, ROLL IT, IT'S TIME TO TOKE.
ONE ADVENTURE GOES MY HEAD
HAVE THE MUNCHIES MAKE A SPREAD
MY BODY IS FLOATING THIS AIN'T NO JOKE.

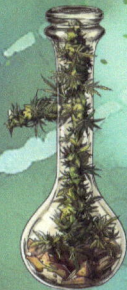

MANNY WAS LAZY AND LOVED TO SLACK.
HIS GIRLFRIEND AND HIM DABBLED IN SMACK.
HE ALWAYS HAS HAD WEED IN HIS BRAIN
AS HE WATCHED DISASTER SHOWS AND LIKE TO EXPLAIN.
HOW SKINNY PEOPLE ARE FAT PEOPLE ON CRACK.

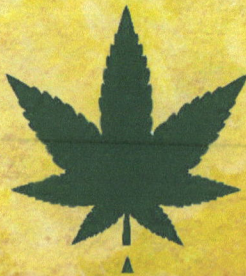

RED SPOOLS
OF THREAD TIED TO
DOORKNOB THAT'S IN HEAVEN
A TOOTHLESS ELF PUCKERS LIPS WITH
LEMONS.

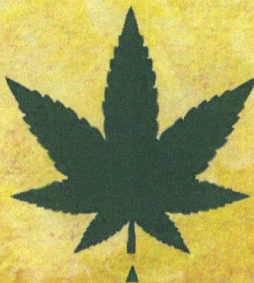

MORNINGS
OF SOME RELIEF
EATING ICE CREAM NOT BEETS.
FORGETTING TO THOROUGHLY COOK
YOUR MEAT.

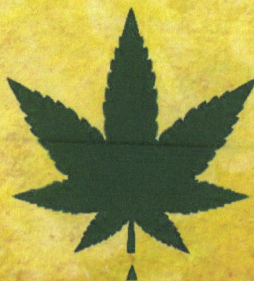

DRAGONS
FLAPPING THEIR WINGS
A HOOKER IN BLUE JEANS
A WRITER'S SPLIFF INTOXICATES
EACH BEAT.

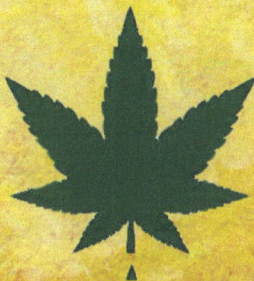

BURNING
MARY'S CHERRY
TRAILS SO GODDAMN WISPY.
ROACHES CAME AFTER JANE BECAME
ASHES.

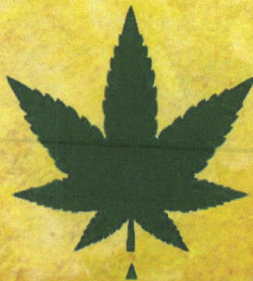

MOON ROCKS
ARE A BLAZING
A RASTA IN TRAINING
YA MON ME DREADS LOOK JUST LIKE BOB
MARLEYS.

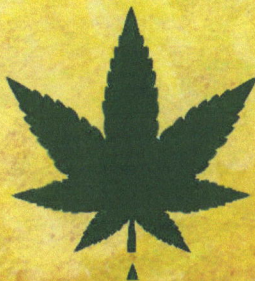

BLUE WAVES
IN A OFFICE
WATCHING THEM TO ESCAPE
AFTER MANY BOWLS OF WEDDING
CAKE SHAKE.

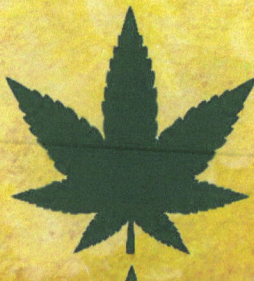

PISTILS
START TO APPEAR
AS LITTLE WHITE HAIRS NOW.
FAN LEAVES GIVING COLAS MUCH NEEDED
AIR NOW.

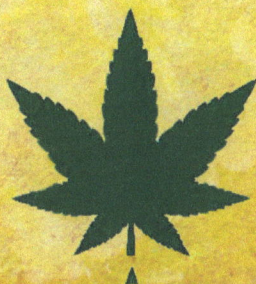

POLKA
DOTTED DREAMS PLAYING
ON AN OLD PHONOGRAPH A MOUSE
DANCING.

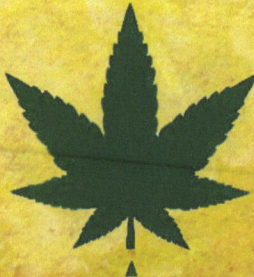

**WELCOME
TO A GREEN WORLD.
CURING OF YOUR MIND IS
AN INHALE AWAY A DREAM THAT
WONT SLEEP.**

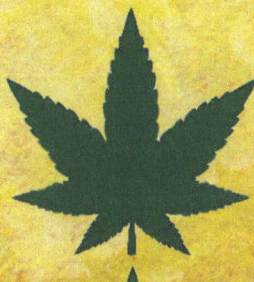

WISPY
TRAILS FOLLOWING
WRINKLED FINGERS HOLDING
ON FOR DEAR LIFE IN BETWEEEN SUCH
LAUGHTER.

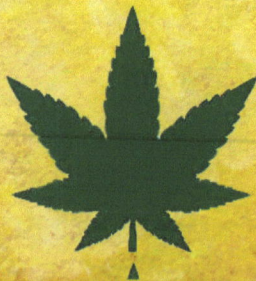

MORNINGS
SUDDENLY CHANGE
LIKE WHEN DOUGH BECOMES BREAD
A CEILING FAN SPINS ABOVE SOME
DEAD HEADS.

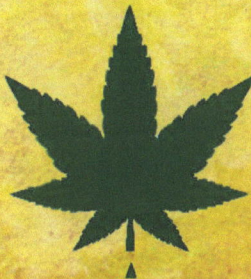

SOMETIMES
SHE SINGS, SOMETIMES
SHE DANCES, SOMETIMES SHE
OPENS LOCKED DOORWAYS. MINDS WELCOME
MARY JANE.

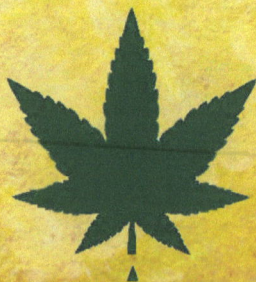

PARCHED LIPS
FLAKE COVERED SHIRTS
DRINKING THAT AWFUL SQUIRT
A VW BUS CHASES JERRY
AROUND.

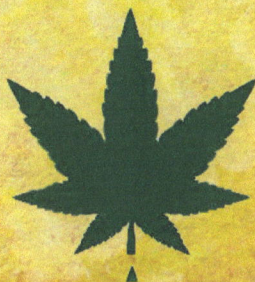

HOTDOGS
AND CHEAP PIZZA
WITH SOME KIND OF COWS MILK
LATE NIGHT STONERS WILL EAT ANY
DAMN THING.

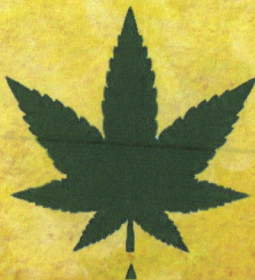

PURPLE
LIGHTS ACROSS FIELDS
GLOWING HORIZON SPEAKS
A MUSHROOMS LANGUAGE NEEDS TONGUES OF
SILVER.

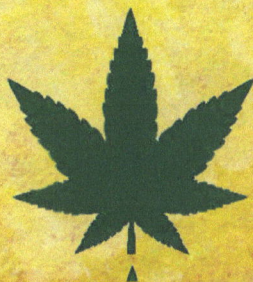

BRING WARMTH
TAKE AWAY TEARS
FROM A HISORY BOOK
ENJOY THE GIFTS FROM LOSING ALL
ANGER.

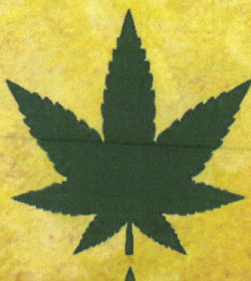

ENJOY
ALL OF THESE CLOUDS
AS THE RIDE NOW BEGINS.
A JOINT SLOWLY BURNS TOWARDS THE
HEAVENS.

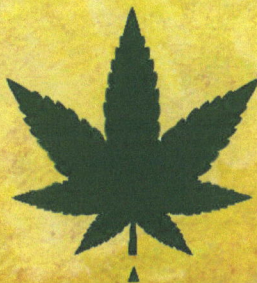

PATTERNS
OF AN OLD CHAIR
APPEAR ON A CLOSET.
TRAILS LEADING TOWARDS A COWBOY
CIRCUS.

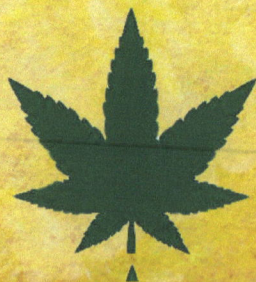

BREAKFAST
NEVER TASTES
QUITE THE SAME AS COTTONMOUTHS
DIFFERENTIATE ALL THE FLAVORS WHILE
SO STONED.

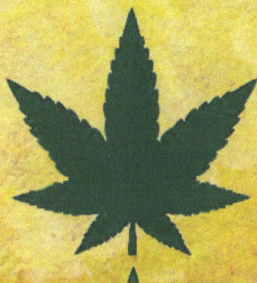

JIMI
PLAYS IN BACKGROUND
ROLLING PAPERS IN HAND
PURPLE HAZE BURNS ÌN EVERY BOWL
PLEASANT.

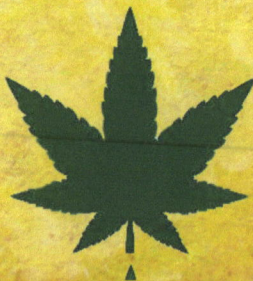

IS THERE
A DIFFERENCE
IN THE FEELINGS NOW MADE
A PERSON BORN TWENTY YEARS TOO
DAMN LATE

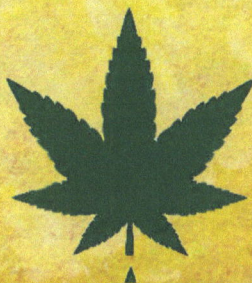

RABBIT
IN A TUNNEL
FLEEING REALITY
TRAILS OF JERRYS CONCERT FOLLOW
THEM HOME.

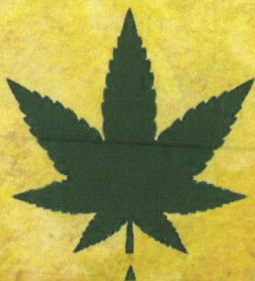

MANY
MEMORIES OF
SUCH SEEDS AND STEMS, COLAS
SMASHED IN TO LITTLE BRICKS WE BOUGHT
LIKE GOLD.

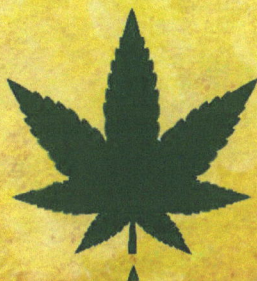

SLEEPING
AFTER WAKING
AND BAKING SOME BROWNIES.
FORGETTING WHAT HAPPENS AFTER
BREAKFAST.

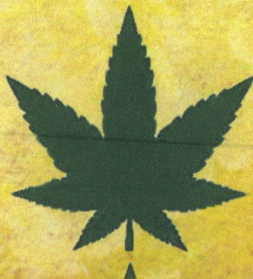

WATCHING
THE WORLD THROUGH A
KALEIDOSCOPE, COLORS
ROTATING TO THE BEAT OF SOME
MUSIC.

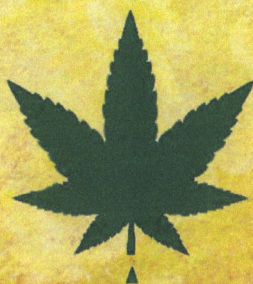

PETER PETER THE FUCKING PUMPKIN EATER
HE LIED ABOUT HIS DIET AND NOW A CHEATER.
COULDN'T RESIST ALL THE MUNCHIES
AND THE M AND MS FILLING OUR BELLIES.
AND HOT DOGS AS LONG AS A METER.

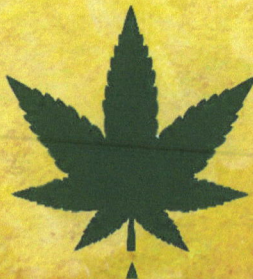

CHOCOLATE BUNNY
HIDDEN QUITE CAREFULLY
AFRAID OF MUNCHIES.

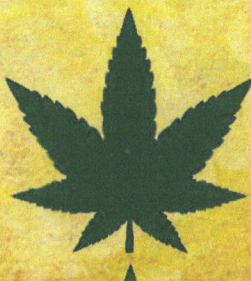

AUTUMN HAS ARRIVED
FLOWERS HANGING UPSIDE DOWN
PLASTIC BAGS READY.

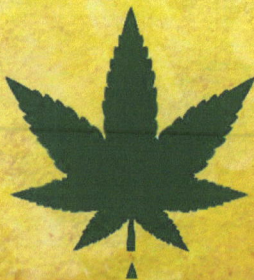

BRAVING HAZY DAYS
BLOOD SHOT EYES SCANNING MENUS
VOLKSWAGON IDLES.

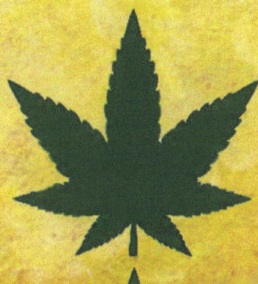

POTATO LISTENS
TO THE GRINDER, JIMI PLAYING.
PAPERS ARE TWISTING.

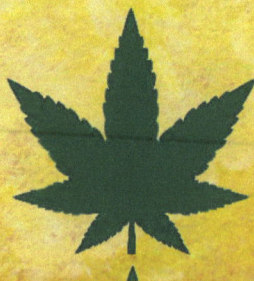

FOLLOW THE BALLONS
CONGREGATE AROUND VOLKSWAGENS
MAYBE EVEN SHROOMS.

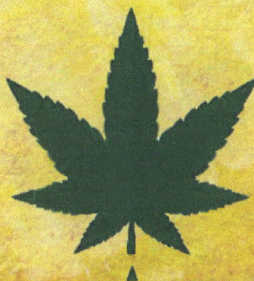

BOWL AFTER BOWL
AFGHAN KUSH STARTS TO BELLOW
EYELIDS ARE DROOPING.

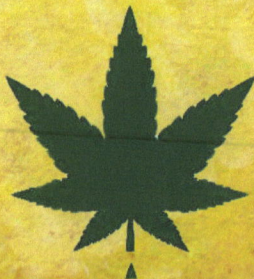

SMOKE FILLING THE ROOM
CASUAL LAUGHTER ECHOES
A JOINT CIRCLES US.

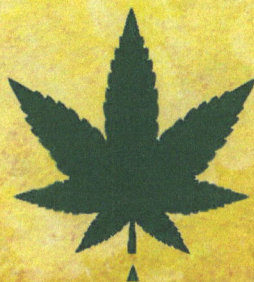

CARAMEL DRIPPING
BANANA SPLIT SUNDAE SHEDS
ALL HER CALORIES.

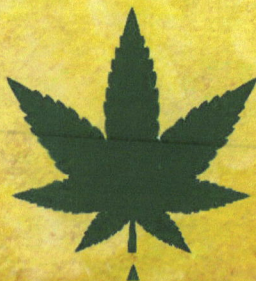

THE KIDS OF TODAY
COMPLAINING ABOUT THE SEEDS
IN OUR OLD BRICK WEED.

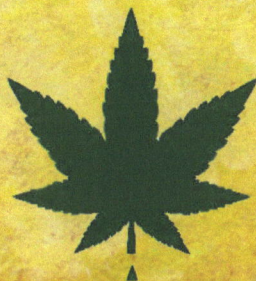

CASUAL SMOKING
RECREATION, MEDICINE?
SHARING LITTLE TREES.

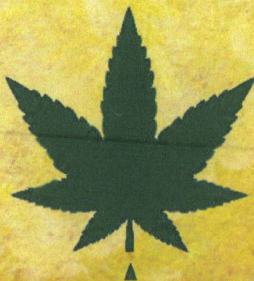

MOTHER IS PLAYING
COUCH POTATO STARTS SINGING
HIGHEST TUNES WELCOME.

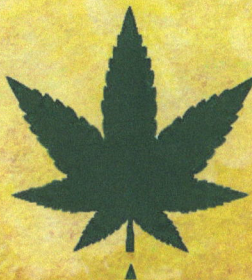

BURNING OUT DAILY
FORGETTING ANY REASONS
I'M FINALLY CLEANSED.

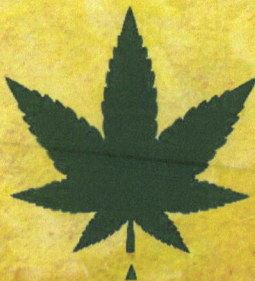

LOOK PIGS ON THE WING
SMOKING ON A TRAMPOLINE
BOUNCY BUZZING TREAT.

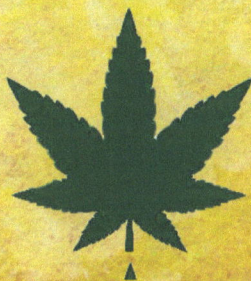

I TRIED TO FIT IN.
BUDS COVERING MANY SCREENS.
DESTINY BURNING.

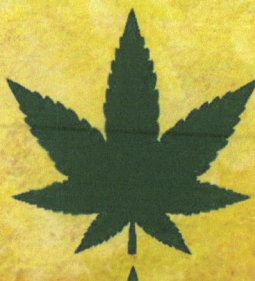

A SCHOOL BELL RINGS
SINGLE CAR PARKED DOWN THE STREET.
ONE LAST PUFF THEN LEAVE.

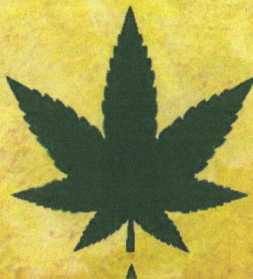

HELLO COTTONMOUTH
HELLO TO THE DANCING BEARS
SMOKING WITH JERRY.

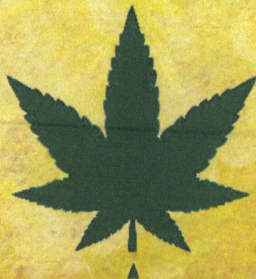

BURNING THE BRAAI WOOD
PASSING OUT THE PREROLLS
SMOKING BOTH ALL DAY.

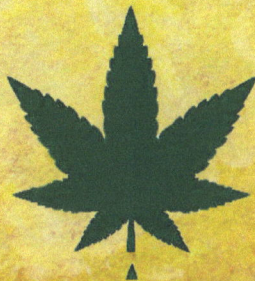

ISLAND ADVENTURES
COFFEE, WEED AND SOME REGGAE
TOURISTS NOW ASLEEP.

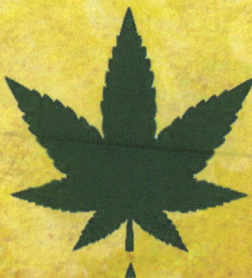

REMEMBER THE DAYS
HANGING AROUND THE MIRRORS
JUST IN CASE ROACH CLIP.

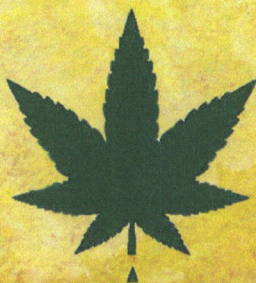

BUBBLING WATER BONGS
DANCING LIGHTS AND LOUD MUSIC
HIGH WITH UNCLE JOHN.

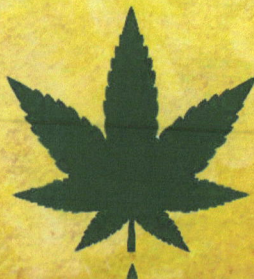

FREEDOM OF THE PRESS
CONCENTRATED FLAVORS TELL
MANY ROSIN TALES.

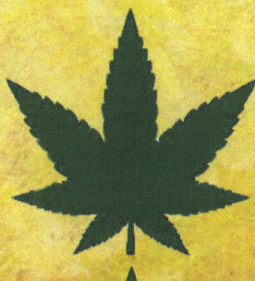

COLORFUL RASTAS
INTERACTING WITH TOURISTS
SELLING THEM SOME WEED.

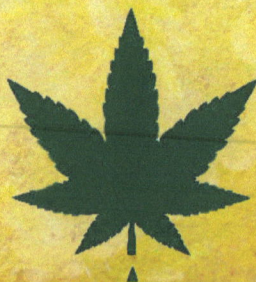

FLOATING WITH THE KITES.
EATING EVERY DAMN THING NOW
TRYING NOT TO SLEEP.

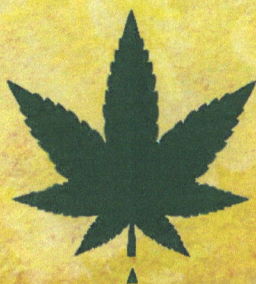

SORTING OUT THE SEEDS
TRIMMING AWAY ALL THE LEAVES
BEFORE THE DRYING.

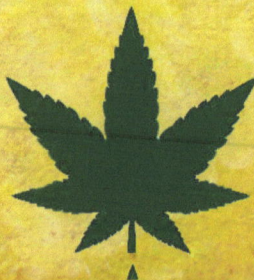

BAGS FILLED WITH SKUNK
PACKED AWAY IN THE TRUNK.
PARANOID DRIVING.

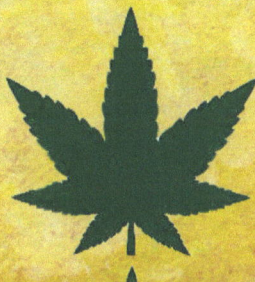

OLD MAN ROCKING ON HIS PORCH
HAS A JOINT IN HAND WITH NO TORCH.
LOOKING TO GET HIGH.
NEEDS MORE STIMULI.
IN SEARCH OF A LIGHTER TO GET SCORCHED.

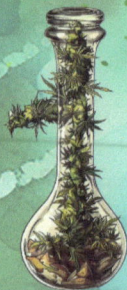

BOWL PACKED
NICE DEEP INHALE
EXHALED SMOKE SWIRLS AROUND ROOM
A BRIEF EPISODE OF COUGHING
HIGHNESS.

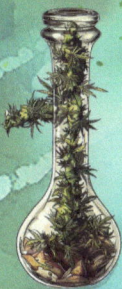

THE WEED CHRONICLES
JOGGING FOGGY MEMORIES OF
YOUTH WITH GREEN.

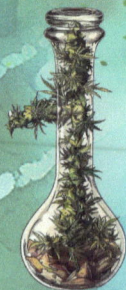

FIRST TIME WITH KIND BUD
A HYDROPONIC LEVEL
A NEW REALM WELCOMED.

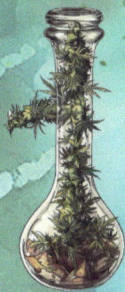

ARCHAIC WEED LAWS
HOW MANY LEGAL STATES NOW?
NO REEFER MADNESS.

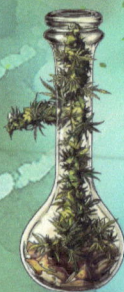

SUNDAY AFTERNOON
TIME TO STRIKE UP AND GET BLAZED
LOVE SELF THERAPY.

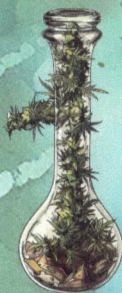

BONG COOL DOWN TECHNIQUE
TRYING SNOW INSTEAD OF ICE
SOUNDS OF BREAKING GLASS
FILL THE STUDIO AGAIN
WHY CAN'T WE LEAVE THINGS AS IS?

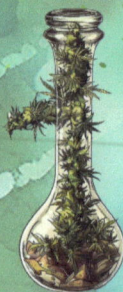

BOWL ALREADY PACKED
MUSIC SET TO THE RIGHT TUNES
I NEEDED TO BUY
THE LIGHTER I FORGOT TO
REMIND MYSELF EARLIER.

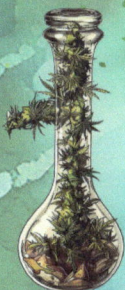

BUTANE TORCH IN HAND
PLANT MATERIAL COMBUSTS
DEEP CHERRY RED HUES

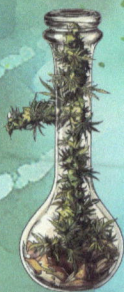

NOSTRILS

FLARED WITH WEED SMOKE

LOOKED IN THE MIRROR

SINCE I'M HIGH, THINKING IT LOOKS COOL

FOOLED.

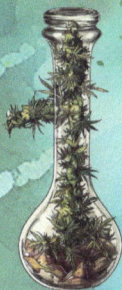

THAT TASTED DIFFERENT
PARANOIA HAS SET IN
WHAT DID I JUST HIT?

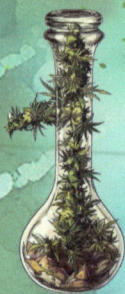

AN URBAN WEED SPOT
FRESH KNOWLEDGE LEARNED FROM COLLEGE
INTIMIDATED.

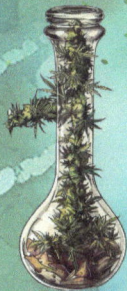

IN TIMES OF NICKELS
AND DIMES NEED TO FIND THE CHANGE
TO SCORE GREENERY.

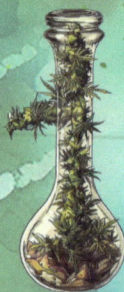

REFLECTED EYE WHITES
BLOOD SHOT AND NO LONGER CLEAR
VISINE HUNT ENSUES

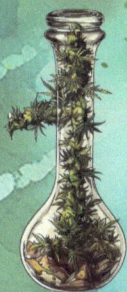

CREATIVITY
HAS SPARKED LIKE A FLAME TO WEED
INHALE THE PROCESS

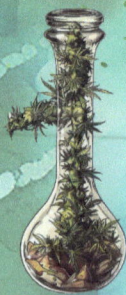

YOU LIKE THE EDIBLES?
REMEMBER PATIENCE IS KEY
ARE THESE WORKING YET?

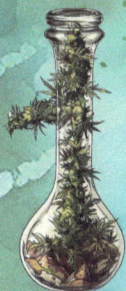

VISITING FAMILY
DISPENSARY SHOP NEEDED
SOME EDIBLES PLEASE.

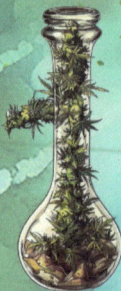

NEVER LOVED FLYING
GONNA EAT A FEW GUMMIES
HOPEFULLY WILL EASE.
THE ANXIETY ABOUT
TO SET IN OR MAYBE NOT.

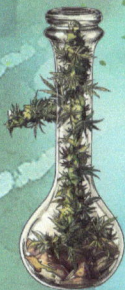

HOME MADE BAKING GOODS
TINTED GREEN COOKIES FROM FRIENDS
BLAST OFF TO THE MOON.

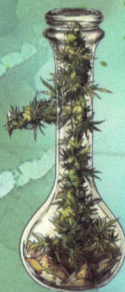

FAMILY OF MY FRIEND
INVITE FOR DINNER AND SMOKE
CAUGHT BY SURPRISE
HOW ACTUALLY HIGH I AM
TRUTH SERUM ACTIVATED.

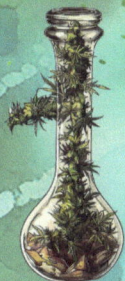

SLOW DOWN THE CHATTER
THAT LIE DEEP INSIDE MY HEAD
LOVE GREEN MEDICINE.

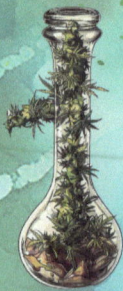

SOUNDS OF THE OCEAN
JOINT IN HAND WITH WAVES CRESTING
ORGANIC ZEN TIME.

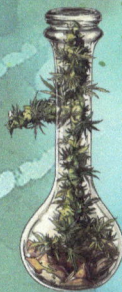

SNOW MOUNTAIN RETREAT
INTRODUCED TO NORTHERN LIGHTS
DIFFICULT TO SKI.

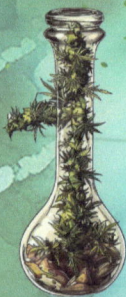

SMILING GIDDINESS
MARY JANE AND I DATING
NEVER FELT LIKE THIS.

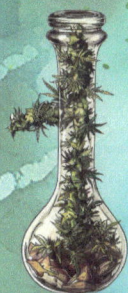

A GENEROUS PLANT
NONSTOP BENEFITS FOR ALL
WE CAN LEARN SO MUCH.

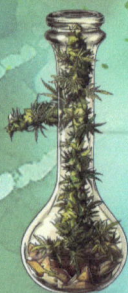

IT'S NOT FOR US ALL
YET NUMEROUS BENEFIT
SHARE SOME WITH A FRIEND.

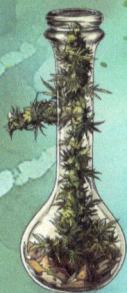

Designed and Published by Sakura Book Publishing
sakurabookpublishing.com

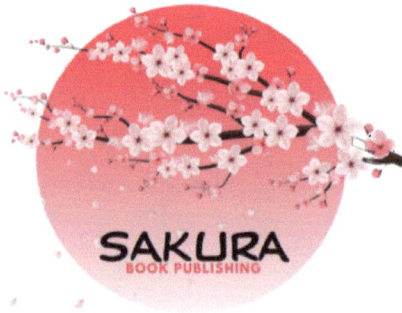

www.ingramcontent.com/pod-product-compliance
Lightning Source LLC
Chambersburg PA
CBHW040931030426
42334CB00007B/116

* 9 7 8 0 7 9 6 1 8 4 9 6 2 *